Healthy People 2020 Topic Areas

1. **Access to Health Services**
2. **Adolescent Health**
3. Arthritis, Osteoporosis, and Chronic Back Conditions
4. Blood Disorders and Blood Safety
5. Cancer
6. Chronic Kidney Disease
7. Dementias, including Alzheimer's Disease
8. Diabetes
9. Disability and Health
10. Early and Middle Childhood
11. **Educational and Community-Based Programs**
12. Environmental Health
13. **Family Planning**
14. Food Safety
15. Genomics
16. Global Health
17. Health Communication and Health Information Technology
18. Healthcare-Associated Infections
19. Health-Related Quality of Life & Well Being
20. Hearing and Other Sensory or Communication Disorders
21. Heart Disease and Stroke
22. **HIV**
23. **Immunization and Infectious Diseases**
24. Injury and Violence Prevention
25. Lesbian, Gay, Bisexual, and Transgender Health
26. **Maternal, Infant, and Child Health**
27. Medical Product Safety
28. Mental Health and Mental Disorders
29. Nutrition and Weight Status
30. Occupational Safety and Health
31. Older Adults
32. Oral Health
33. Physical Activity
34. Preparedness
35. Public Health Infrastructure
36. Respiratory Diseases
37. **Sexually Transmitted Diseases**
38. Sleep Health
39. Social Determinants of Health
40. Substance Abuse
41. Tobacco Use
42. Vision

Table of Contents

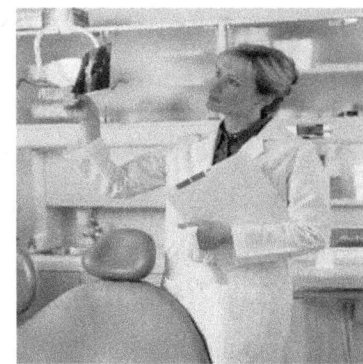

Access to Health Services

Goal
Improve access to comprehensive, quality health care services.

Overview
Access to comprehensive, quality health care services is important for the achievement of health equity and for increasing the quality of a healthy life for everyone. This topic area focuses on four components of access to care: coverage, services, timeliness, and workforce.

Why Is Access to Health Services Important?
Access to health services means the timely use of personal health services to achieve the best health outcomes.[1] It requires three distinct steps:
(1)   gaining entry into the health care system;
(2)   accessing a health care location where needed services are provided; and
(3)   finding a health care provider with whom the patient can communicate and trust.[2]

Access to health care impacts:
- Overall physical, social, and mental health status;
- Prevention of disease and disability;
- Detection and treatment of health conditions;
- Quality of life;
- Preventable death; and
- Life expectancy.

The Reproductive Health-Related Objective(s) are listed below.

- **AHS-1 Increase the proportion of persons with health insurance.**

Data Source:	National Health Interview Survey (NHIS), CDC, NCHS
Baseline:	83.2 percent of persons had medical insurance in 2008
Target:	100 percent
Target-Setting Methodology:	Total coverage

Access to Health Services

- **AHS-2 (Developmental)* Increase the proportion of insured persons with coverage for clinical preventive services.**

Data Source:	Children's Health Insurance Program (CHIP), CMS; AGing Integrated Database (AGID), AoA; CMS claims data and Medicare Current Beneficiary Survey (MCBS), CMS
Baseline:	TBD
Target:	TBD
Target-Setting Methodology:	TBD

* Developmental objectives currently do not have national baseline data but address subjects of sufficient national importance that inclusion on the national agenda for data collection is warranted. Investments should be made over the next decade to measure their change.

Adolescent Health

Goal
Improve the healthy development, health, safety, and well-being of adolescents and young adults.

Overview
Adolescents (ages 10 to 19) and young adults (ages 20 to 24) make up 21 percent of the population of the United States.[3] The behavioral patterns established during these developmental periods help determine young people's current health status and their risk for developing chronic diseases in adulthood.[4]

Although adolescence and young adulthood are generally healthy times of life, several important public health and social problems either peak or start during these years. Because they are in developmental transition, adolescents and young adults are particularly sensitive to environmental—that is, contextual or surrounding—influences.[5] Environmental factors, including family, peer group, school, neighborhood, policies, and societal cues, can either support or challenge young people's health and well-being.[6] Addressing the positive development of young people facilitates their adoption of healthy behaviors and helps to ensure a healthy and productive future adult population.[7]

Why Is Adolescent Health Important?
Adolescence is a critical transitional period that includes the biological changes of puberty and the need to negotiate key developmental tasks, such as increasing independence and normative experimentation.[5, 7, 8]

The Reproductive Health-Related Objective(s) are listed below.

- **AH-3 Increase the proportion of adolescents who are connected to a parent or other positive adult caregiver.**

    - **AH-3.1 Increase the proportion of adolescents who have an adult in their lives with whom they can talk about serious problems.**

Data Source:	National Survey on Drug Use and Health (NSDUH), SAMHSA
Baseline:	75.7 percent of adolescents aged 12 to 17 years had an adult in their lives with whom they could talk about serious problems, as reported in 2008
Target:	83.3 percent
Target-Setting Methodology:	10 percent improvement

Educational and Community-Based Programs

Goal
Increase the quality, availability, and effectiveness of educational and community-based programs designed to prevent disease and injury, improve health, and enhance quality of life.

Overview
Educational and community-based programs play a key role in:

- Preventing disease and injury;
- Improving health; and
- Enhancing quality of life.

Health status and related health behaviors are determined by influences at multiple levels: personal, organizational/institutional, environmental, and policy. Because significant and dynamic interrelationships exist among these different levels of health determinants, educational and community-based programs are most likely to succeed in improving health and wellness when they address influences at all levels and in a variety of environments/settings.

Why Are Educational and Community-Based Programs Important?
Educational and community-based programs and strategies played an important role in reaching Healthy People 2010 objectives. Over the next decade, they will continue to contribute to the improvement of health outcomes in the United States.

Educational and community-based programs and strategies are designed to reach people outside of traditional health care settings. These settings may include:

- Schools;
- Worksites;
- Health care facilities; and
- Communities.

Each setting provides opportunities to reach people using existing social structures. This maximizes impact and reduces the time and resources necessary for program development. People often have high levels of contact with these settings, both directly and indirectly. Programs that combine multiple—if not all 4—settings can have a greater impact than programs using only 1 setting. While populations reached will sometimes overlap, people who are not accessible in 1 setting may be in another.[9]

Using nontraditional settings can help encourage informal information sharing within communities through peer social interaction. Reaching out to people in different settings also allows for greater tailoring of health information and education.

Educational and Community-Based Programs

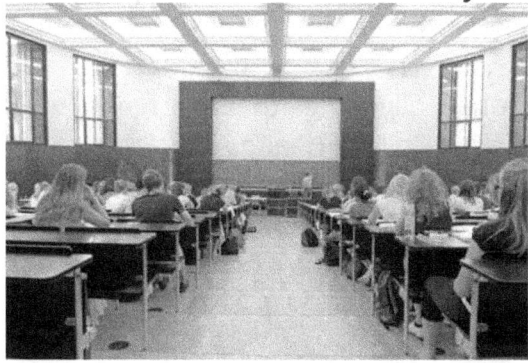

The Reproductive Health-Related Objective(s) are listed below.

- **ECBP-2: Increase the proportion of elementary, middle, and senior high schools that provide comprehensive school health education to prevent health problems in the following areas: unintentional injury; violence; suicide; tobacco use and addiction; alcohol or other drug use; unintended pregnancy; HIV/AIDS and STD infection; unhealthy dietary patterns; and inadequate physical activity.**

    - **ECBP-2.7 Unintended pregnancy, HIV/AIDS, and STD infection**

Data Source:	School Health Policies and Programs Study (SHPPS), CDC, NCCDPHP
Baseline:	39.3 percent of elementary, middle, and senior high schools provide comprehensive school health education to prevent unintended pregnancy, HIV/AIDS and STD infection in 2006
Target:	43.2 percent
Target-Setting Methodology:	10 percent improvement

- **ECBP-7 Increase the proportion of college and university students who receive information from their institution on each of the priority health risk behavior areas (all priority areas; unintentional injury; violence; suicide; tobacco use and addiction; alcohol and other drug use; unintended pregnancy, HIV/AIDS, and STD infection; unhealthy dietary patterns; and inadequate physical activity).**

    - **ECBP-7.7 Unintended pregnancy**

Data Source:	National College Health Assessment, American College Health Association
Baseline:	39.9 percent of college and university students received health-risk behavior information on unintended pregnancy from their institution in 2009
Target:	43.9 percent
Target-Setting Methodology:	10 percent improvement

Educational and Community-Based Programs

- ○ **ECBP-7.8 HIV, AIDS and STD infection**
  - Data Source: National College Health Assessment, American College Health Association
  - Baseline: 52.5 percent of college and university students received health-risk behavior information on HIV/AIDS and STD infection from their institution in 2009
  - Target: 57.8 percent
  - Target-Setting Methodology: 10 percent improvement

- **ECBP-10 Increase the number of community-based organizations (including local health departments, tribal health services, nongovernmental organizations, and State agencies) providing population-based primary prevention services in the following areas:**

  - ○ **ECBP-10.6. Unintended pregnancy.**
    - Data Source: National Profile of Local Health Departments, National Association of County and City Health Officials (NACCHO)
    - Baseline: 81.3 percent of community-based organizations (including local health departments, tribal health services, nongovernmental organizations, and State agencies) provided population-based primary prevention services in unintended pregnancy in 2008
    - Target: 89.4 percent
    - Target-Setting Methodology: 10 percent improvement

Family Planning

Goal
Improve pregnancy planning and spacing, and prevent unintended pregnancy.

Overview
Family planning is one of the ten great public health achievements of the 20th century.[10] The availability of family planning services allows individuals to achieve desired birth spacing and family size and contributes to improved health outcomes for infants, children, and women.[10]

Family planning services include:
- Contraceptive and broader reproductive health services, including patient education and counseling;
- Breast and pelvic examinations;
- Breast and cervical cancer screening;
- Sexually transmitted infection (STI) and human immunodeficiency virus (HIV) prevention education, counseling, testing, and referral; and
- Pregnancy diagnosis and counseling.[11, 12, 13]

Abstinence from sexual activity is the only 100 percent effective way to avoid unintended pregnancy. For individuals who are sexually active, correct and consistent contraceptive use during every act of sexual intercourse is effective at preventing unintended pregnancy. Condom use is the only contraceptive method that protects against both unintended pregnancy and sexually transmitted infections (STIs); men and women should be encouraged to use condoms in addition to a long-acting, reversible contraceptive method at every act of sexual intercourse.

Why Is Family Planning Important?
For many women, a family planning clinic is their entry point into the health care system and is considered to be their usual source of care.[11, 14] This is especially true for women with incomes below 100 percent of the poverty level, women who are uninsured, Hispanic women, and black women.[14] Each year, publicly funded family planning services prevent 1.94 million unintended pregnancies, including 400,000 teen pregnancies.[12] These services are highly cost-effective, saving $4 for every $1 spent.[15]

Unintended pregnancies are associated with many negative health and economic outcomes. Unintended pregnancies include pregnancies that are reported by women as being mistimed or unwanted. In 2001, almost half of all pregnancies in the United States were unintended.[16] The rate of unintended pregnancies declined significantly between 1987 and 1994; however, since then, the rate has remained stable.[16] The direct medical costs associated with unintended pregnancies in 2002 were $5 billion, or an average of $1,609 for each unintended pregnancy.[17]

For women, negative outcomes associated with unintended pregnancy include:
- delays in initiating prenatal care;

Family Planning

- reduced likelihood of breastfeeding;
- poor maternal mental health;
- lower mother-child relationship quality; and
- increased risk of physical violence during pregnancy.[18, 19, 20, 21]

The Reproductive Health-Related Objective(s) are listed below.

- **FP-1 Increase the proportion of pregnancies that are intended.**

Data Source:	National Survey of Family Growth (NSFG), CDC, NCHS; National Vital Statistics System (NVSS), CDC, NCHS; Abortion Provider Survey, Guttmacher Institute; Abortion Surveillance Data, CDC, NCCDPHP
Baseline:	51.0 percent of all pregnancies were intended, as reported in 2002
Target:	56.0 percent
Target-Setting Methodology:	10 percent improvement

- **FP-2 Reduce the proportion of females experiencing pregnancy despite use of a reversible contraceptive method.**

Data Source:	National Survey of Family Growth (NSFG), CDC, NCHS; Abortion Provider Survey, Guttmacher Institute
Baseline:	12.4 percent of females experienced pregnancy despite use of a reversible contraceptive method, as reported in 2002
Target:	9.9 percent
Target-Setting Methodology:	20 percent improvement based on trend analysis

- **FP-3 Increase the proportion of publicly funded family planning clinics that offer the full-range of FDA-approved methods of contraception, including emergency contraception, onsite.**

  - **FP-3.1 Increase the proportion of publicly funded family planning clinics that offer the full range of FDA-approved methods of contraception onsite.**

Data Source:	Survey of Contraceptive Service Providers, Guttmacher Institute
Baseline:	38.3 percent of publicly funded family planning clinics offered the full range of FDA-approved methods of contraception onsite, as reported in 2003
Target:	47.9 percent
Target-Setting Methodology:	25 percent improvement

Family Planning

- **FP-3.2 Increase the proportion of publicly funded family planning clinics that offer emergency contraception onsite.**

Data Source:	Survey of Contraceptive Service Providers, Guttmacher Institute
Baseline:	79.7 percent of publicly funded family planning clinics offered emergency contraception onsite, as reported in 2003
Target:	87.7 percent
Target-Setting Methodology:	10 percent improvement

- **FP-4 (Developmental) Increase the proportion of health insurance plans that cover contraceptive supplies and services.**

Data Source:	Guttmacher Institute
Baseline:	TBD
Target:	TBD
Target-Setting Methodology:	TBD

- **FP-5 Reduce the proportion of pregnancies conceived within 18 months of a previous birth.**

Data Source:	National Survey of Family Growth, CDC, NCHS
Baseline:	35.3 percent of pregnancies were conceived within 18 months of a previous birth, as reported in 2006-8
Target:	31.7 percent
Target-Setting Methodology:	10 percent improvement

- **FP-6 Increase the proportion of females or their partners at risk of unintended pregnancy who used contraception at most recent sexual intercourse.**

Data Source:	National Survey of Family Growth (NSFG), CDC, NCHS
Baseline:	83.0 percent of females or their partners at risk of unintended pregnancy used contraception at most recent sexual intercourse, as reported in 2006-8
Target:	91.3 percent
Target-Setting Methodology:	10 percent improvement

Family Planning

- **FP-7 Increase the proportion of sexually active persons who received reproductive health services.**

  - **FP-7.1 Increase the proportion of sexually active females aged 15 to 44 years who received reproductive health services.**

    Data Source: National Survey of Family Growth (NSFG), CDC, NCHS

    Baseline: 78.8 percent of sexually active females aged 15 to 44 years received reproductive health services in the past 12 months, as reported in 2006-8

    Target: 86.7 percent

    Target-Setting Methodology: 10 percent improvement

  - **FP-7.2 Increase the proportion of sexually active males aged 15 to 44 years who received reproductive health services.**

    Data Source: National Survey of Family Growth (NSFG), CDC, NCHS

    Baseline: 14.9 percent of sexually active males aged 15 to 44 years received reproductive health services in the past 12 months, as reported in 2006-08

    Target: 16.4 percent

    Target-Setting Methodology: 10 percent improvement

- **FP-8 Reduce pregnancy rates among adolescent females.**

  - **FP-8.1 Reduce the pregnancy rate among adolescent females aged 15 to 17 years.**

    Data Source: Abortion Provider Survey, Guttmacher Institute; Abortion Surveillance Data, CDC, NCCDPHP; National Vital Statistics System–Natality (NVSS–N), CDC, NCHS; National Survey of Family Growth (NSFG), CDC, NCHS

    Baseline: 40.2 pregnancies per 1,000 females aged 15 to 17 years occurred in 2005

    Target: 36.2 pregnancies per 1,000

    Target-Setting Methodology: 10 percent improvement

Family Planning

- o **FP-8.2 Reduce the pregnancy rate among adolescent females aged 18 to 19 years.**

Data Source:	Abortion Provider Survey, Guttmacher Institute; National Vital Statistics System (NVSS), CDC, NCHS; National Survey of Family Growth (NSFG), CDC, NCHS; Abortion Surveillance Data, CDC, NCCDPHP
Baseline:	117.7 pregnancies per 1,000 females aged 18 to 19 years occurred in 2005
Target:	105.9 pregnancies per 1,000
Target-Setting Methodology:	10 percent improvement

Family Planning

- **FP-9: Increase the proportion of adolescents aged 17 years and under who have never had sexual intercourse.**

    - **FP-9.1 Female adolescents aged 15 to 17 years**

Data Source:	National Survey of Family Growth (NSFG), CDC, NCHS
Baseline:	72.1 percent of female adolescents aged 15 to 17 years reported they had never had sexual intercourse in 2006-8
Target:	79.3 percent
Target-Setting Methodology:	10 percent improvement

    - **FP-9.2 Male adolescents aged 15 to 17 years**

Data Source:	National Survey of Family Growth (NSFG), CDC, NCHS
Baseline:	71.2 percent of male adolescents aged 15 to 17 years reported they had never had sexual intercourse in 2006-8
Target:	78.3 percent
Target-Setting Methodology:	10 percent improvement

    - **FP-9.3 Female adolescents aged 15 years and under**

Data Source:	National Survey of Family Growth (NSFG), CDC, NCHS
Baseline:	82.9 percent of female adolescents aged 15 years had never had sexual intercourse, as reported in 2006-8
Target:	91.2 percent
Target-Setting Methodology:	10 percent improvement

    - **FP-9.4 Male adolescents aged 15 years and under**

Data Source:	National Survey of Family Growth (NSFG), CDC
Baseline:	82.0 percent of male adolescents aged 15 years had never had sexual intercourse, as reported in 2006-08
Target:	90.2 percent
Target-Setting Methodology:	10 percent improvement

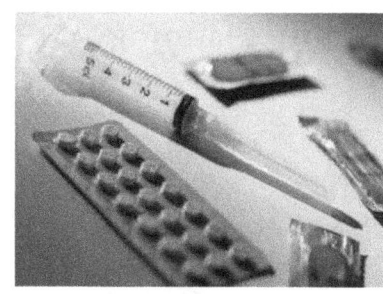

Family Planning

- **FP-10 Increase the proportion of sexually active persons aged 15 to 19 years who use condoms to both effectively prevent pregnancy and provide barrier protection against disease.**

  - **FP-10.1 Increase the proportion of sexually active females aged 15 to 19 years who use a condom at first intercourse.**

Data Source:	National Survey of Family Growth (NSFG), CDC
Baseline:	66.9 percent of sexually active females aged 15 to 19 years used a condom at first intercourse, as reported in 2006–8
Target:	73.6 percent
Target-Setting Methodology:	10 percent improvement

  - **FP-10.2 Increase the proportion of sexually active males aged 15 to 19 years who use a condom at first intercourse**

Data Source:	National Survey of Family Growth (NSFG), CDC
Baseline:	80.6 percent of sexually active males aged 15 to 19 years used a condom at first intercourse as reported in 2006–8
Target:	88.6 percent
Target-Setting Methodology:	10 percent improvement

  - **FP-10.3 Increase the proportion of sexually active females aged 15 to 19 years who use a condom at last intercourse.**

Data Source:	National Survey of Family Growth (NSFG), CDC
Baseline:	52.8 percent of sexually active females aged 15 to 19 years used a condom at last intercourse as reported in 2006–8
Target:	58.1 percent
Target-Setting Methodology:	10 percent improvement

Family Planning

- o **FP-10.4 Increase the proportion of sexually active males aged 15 to 19 years who use a condom at last intercourse.**

Data Source:	National Survey of Family Growth (NSFG), CDC
Baseline:	77.9 percent of sexually active males aged 15 to 19 years used a condom at last intercourse, as reported in 2006–8
Target:	85.7 percent
Target-Setting Methodology:	10 percent improvement

- • **FP-11 Increase the proportion of sexually active persons aged 15 to 19 years who use condoms and hormonal or intrauterine contraception to both effectively prevent pregnancy and provide barrier protection against disease.**

  - o **FP-11.1 Increase the proportion of sexually active females aged 15 to 19 years who use a condom and hormonal or intrauterine contraception at first intercourse.**

Data Source:	National Survey of Family Growth (NSFG), CDC
Baseline:	13.4 percent of sexually active females aged 15 to 19 years used a condom and hormonal or intrauterine contraception at first intercourse as reported in 2006–8
Target:	14.8 percent
Target-Setting Methodology:	10 percent improvement

  - o **FP-11.2 Increase the proportion of sexually active males aged 15 to 19 years who use a condom and hormonal or intrauterine contraception at first intercourse.**

Data Source:	National Survey of Family Growth (NSFG), CDC
Baseline:	18.1 percent of sexually active males aged 15 to 19 years used a condom and hormonal or intrauterine contraception at first intercourse as reported in 2006–8
Target:	19.9 percent
Target-Setting Methodology:	10 percent improvement

Family Planning

- o **FP-11.3 Increase the proportion of sexually active females aged 15 to 19 years who use a condom and hormonal or intrauterine contraception at last intercourse.**

Data Source:	National Survey of Family Growth (NSFG), CDC
Baseline:	18.4 percent of sexually active females aged 15 to 19 years used a condom and hormonal or intrauterine contraception at last intercourse as reported in 2006–8
Target:	20.2 percent
Target-Setting Methodology:	10 percent improvement

- o **FP-11.4 Increase the proportion of sexually active males aged 15 to 19 years who use a condom and hormonal or intrauterine contraception at last intercourse.**

Data Source:	National Survey of Family Growth (NSFG), CDC
Baseline:	33.0 of sexually active males aged 15 to 19 years used a condom and hormonal or intrauterine contraception at last intercourse as reported in 2006–8
Target:	36.3 percent
Target-Setting Methodology:	10 percent improvement

- **FP-12 Increase the proportion of adolescents who received formal instruction on reproductive health topics before they were 18 years old.**

  - o **FP-12.1 Abstinence—females**

Data Source:	National Survey of Family Growth (NSFG), CDC, NCHS
Baseline:	87.2 percent of female adolescents received formal instruction on how to say no to sex before they were 18 years old, as reported in 2006-8
Target:	95.9 percent
Target-Setting Methodology:	10 percent improvement

Family Planning

- ○ **FP-12.2 Abstinence—males**

Data Source:	National Survey of Family Growth (NSFG), CDC, NCHS
Baseline:	81.1 percent of male adolescents received formal instruction on how to say no to sex before they were 18 years old in 2002, as reported in 2006-8
Target:	89.2 percent
Target-Setting Methodology:	10 percent improvement

- ○ **FP-12.3 Birth control methods—females**

Data Source:	National Survey of Family Growth (NSFG), CDC, NCHS
Baseline:	69.5 percent of females received formal instruction on birth control methods before they were 18 years old, as reported in 2006-8
Target:	76.4 percent
Target-Setting Methodology:	10 percent improvement

- ○ **FP-12.4 Birth control methods—males**

Data Source:	National Survey of Family Growth (NSFG), CDC, NCHS
Baseline:	61.9 percent of males received formal instruction on birth control methods before they were 18 years old, as reported in 2006-8
Target:	68.1 percent
Target-Setting Methodology:	10 percent improvement

- ○ **FP-12.5 HIV/AIDS prevention—females**

Data Source:	National Survey of Family Growth (NSFG), CDC, NCHS
Baseline:	88.3 percent of females received formal instruction on HIV/AIDS prevention before they were 18 years old, as reported in 2006-8
Target:	97.2 percent
Target-Setting Methodology:	10 percent improvement

Family Planning

- **FP-12.6 HIV/AIDS prevention—males**

Data Source:	National Survey of Family Growth (NSFG), CDC, NCHS
Baseline:	89.0 percent of males received formal instruction on HIV/AIDS prevention before they were 18 years old, as reported in 2006-8
Target:	97.9 percent
Target-Setting Methodology:	10 percent improvement

- **FP-12.7 Sexually transmitted diseases—females**

Data Source:	National Survey of Family Growth (NSFG), CDC, NCHS
Baseline:	93.2 percent of females received formal instruction on sexually transmitted disease prevention methods before they were 18 years old, as reported in 2006-8
Target:	95.2 percent
Target-Setting Methodology:	2 percentage point improvement

- **FP-12.8 Sexually transmitted diseases—males**

Data Source:	National Survey of Family Growth (NSFG), CDC, NCHS
Baseline:	92.2 percent of males received formal instruction on sexually transmitted disease prevention methods before they were 18 years old, as reported in 2006-8
Target:	94.2 percent
Target-Setting Methodology:	2 percentage point improvement

Family Planning

- **FP-13 Increase the proportion of adolescents who talked to a parent or guardian about reproductive health topics before they were 18 years old.**

    o **FP-13.1 Abstinence—females**

Data Source:	National Survey of Family Growth (NSFG), CDC, NCHS
Baseline:	63.1 percent of female adolescents talked with a parent or guardian about how to say no to sex before they were 18 years old, as reported in 2006-8
Target:	69.4 percent
Target-Setting Methodology:	10 percent improvement

    o **FP-13.2 Abstinence—males**

Data Source:	National Survey of Family Growth (NSFG), CDC, NCHS
Baseline:	41.8 percent of male adolescents talked to a parent or guardian about how to say no to sex before they were 18 years old, as in 2006-8
Target:	5.9 percent
Target-Setting Methodology:	0 percent improvement

    o **FP-13.3 Birth control methods—females**

Data Source:	National Survey of Family Growth (NSFG), CDC, NCHS
Baseline:	50.5 percent of female adolescents talked to a parent or guardian about birth control methods before they were 18 years old, as reported in 2006-8
Target:	55.6 percent
Target-Setting Methodology:	10 percent improvement

Family Planning

- **FP-13.4 Birth control methods—males**

Data Source:	National Survey of Family Growth (NSFG), CDC, NCHS
Baseline:	30.6 percent of male adolescents talked to a parent or guardian about birth control methods before they were 18 years old, as reported in 2006-8
Target:	33.6 percent
Target-Setting Methodology:	10 percent improvement

- **FP-13.5: HIV/AIDS prevention—females**

Data Source:	National Survey of Family Growth (NSFG), CDC, NCHS
Baseline:	55.2 percent of female adolescents talked to a parent or guardian about HIV/AIDS prevention before they were 18 years old, as reported in 2006-8
Target:	60.7 percent
Target-Setting Methodology:	10 percent improvement

- **FP-13.6 HIV/AIDS prevention—males**

Data Source:	National Survey of Family Growth (NSFG), CDC, NCHS
Baseline:	49.3 percent of male adolescents talked to a parent or guardian about HIV/AIDS prevention before they were 18 years old, as reported in 2006-8
Target:	54.3 percent
Target-Setting Methodology:	10 percent improvement

- **FP-13.7 Sexually transmitted diseases—females**

Data Source:	National Survey of Family Growth (NSFG), CDC, NCHS
Baseline:	55.2 percent of female adolescents talked to a parent or guardian about sexually transmitted diseases before they were 18 years old, as reported in 2006-8
Target:	60.7 percent
Target-Setting Methodology:	10 percent improvement

Family Planning

- FP-13.8 **Sexually transmitted diseases—males**

Data Source:	National Survey of Family Growth (NSFG), CDC, NCHS
Baseline:	38.5 percent of male adolescents talked to a parent or guardian about sexually transmitted diseases before they were 18 years old, as reported in 2006-8
Target:	42.3 percent
Target-Setting Methodology:	10 percent improvement

- **FP-14 Increase the number of States that set the income eligibility level for Medicaid-covered family planning services to at least the same level used to determine eligibility for Medicaid-covered, pregnancy-related care.**

Data Source:	Guttmacher Institute, State Medicaid Family Planning Eligibility Expansions—national, State-based data (includes data for all 50 States); State Medicaid Family Planning Eligibility Expansions, Guttmacher Institute; Medicaid Income Eligibility Levels for Pregnant Women, Kaiser Family Foundation—national, State-based data (includes data for all 50 States)
Baseline:	21 states set the income eligibility level for Medicaid-covered family planning services to at least the same level used to determine eligibility for Medicaid-covered, pregnancy-related care in 2010
Target:	32 States
Target-Setting Methodology:	Trend analysis

- **FP-15 Increase the proportion of females in need of publicly supported contraceptive services and supplies who receive those services and supplies.**

Data Source:	Contraceptive Needs and Services, Guttmacher Institute
Baseline:	53.8 percent of females in need of publicly supported contraceptive services and supplies reported receiving those services and supplies in 2006
Target:	64.5 percent
Target-Setting Methodology:	20 percent improvement

Human Immunodefiency Virus (HIV) Infection

Goal
Prevent human immunodeficiency virus (HIV) infection and its related illness and death.

Overview
The HIV epidemic in the United States continues to be a major public health crisis. An estimated 1.1 million Americans are living with HIV, and one out of five people with HIV do not know they are infected with it.[22] HIV continues to spread, leading to about 56,000 new HIV infections each year.[23]

In 2010, the White House released a National HIV/AIDS Strategy. The strategy includes three primary goals:

- Reducing the number of people who become infected with HIV;
- Increasing access to care and improving health outcomes for people living with HIV; and
- Reducing HIV-related health disparities.

Why Is HIV Important?
HIV is a preventable disease. Effective HIV prevention interventions have been proven to reduce HIV transmission. People who get tested for HIV and learn that they are infected can make significant behavior changes to improve their health and reduce the risk of transmitting HIV to their sex or drug-using partners. More than 50 percent of new HIV infections[24] occur as a result of the 21 percent of people who have HIV but do not know it.

The Reproductive Health-Related Objective(s) are:

- **HIV-2 (Developmental) Reduce new (incident) HIV infections among adolescents and adults.**
Data Source:	HIV Surveillance System, CDC, NCHHSTP
Baseline:	TBD
Target:	TBD
Target-Setting Methodology:	TBD

- **HIV-13 Increase the proportion of people living with HIV who know their serostatus.**
Data Source:	HIV Surveillance System, CDC, NCHHSTP
Baseline:	79.0 percent of persons aged 13 years and older living with HIV were aware of their HIV infection in 2006
Target:	90.0 percent
Target-Setting Methodology:	Consistent with the National HIV Strategy

Human Immunodefiency Virus (HIV) Infection

- **HIV-14 Increase the proportion of adolescents and adults who have been tested for HIV in the past 12 months.**

    - **HIV-14.1 Adolescents and adults**

Data Source:	National Survey of Family Growth (NSFG), CDC, NCHS
Baseline:	15.4 percent of persons 15-44 years of age reported that they had an HIV test in the past 12 months, outside of blood donation in 2006-8
Target:	16.9 percent
Target-Setting Methodology:	10 percent improvement

    - **HIV-14.4 Adolescents and young adults**

Data Source:	National Survey of Family Growth (NSFG), CDC, NCHS
Baseline:	15.6 percent of persons 15 to 24 years of age reported that they had an HIV test in the past 12 months, outside of blood donation in 2006-8
Target:	17.2 percent
Target-Setting Methodology:	10 percent improvement

    - **HIV-17.1 Unmarried females aged 15 to 44 years**

Data Source:	National Survey of Family Growth (NSFG), CDC, NCHS
Baseline:	34.5 percent of sexually active, unmarried females aged 15 to 44 years reported using a condom at last sexual intercourse in 2006-8
Target:	38.0 percent
Target-Setting Methodology:	10 percent improvement

    - **HIV-17.2 Unmarried males aged 15 to 44 years**

Data Source:	National Survey of Family Growth (NSFG), CDC, NCHS
Baseline:	55.2 percent of sexually active, unmarried males aged 15 to 44 years reported using a condom at last sexual intercourse in 2006-8
Target:	60.7 percent
Target-Setting Methodology:	10 percent improvement

Immunization and Infectious Disease

Goal
Increase immunization rates and reduce preventable infectious diseases.

Overview
The increase in life expectancy during the 20th century is largely due to improvements in child survival; this increase is associated with reductions in infectious disease mortality, due largely to immunization.[25] However, infectious diseases remain a major cause of illness, disability, and death. Immunization recommendations in the United States currently target 17 vaccine-preventable diseases across the lifespan.

Healthy People 2020 goals for immunization and infectious diseases (IID) are rooted in evidence-based clinical and community activities and services for the prevention and treatment of infectious diseases. Objectives new to Healthy People 2020 focus on technological advancements and ensuring that States, local public health departments, and nongovernmental organizations are strong partners in the Nation's attempt to control the spread of infectious diseases. Objectives for 2020 reflect a more mobile society and the fact that diseases do not stop at geopolitical borders.

Why Are Immunization and Infectious Diseases Important?
People in the United States continue to get diseases that are vaccine preventable. Viral hepatitis, influenza, and tuberculosis (TB) remain among the leading causes of illness and death in the United States and account for substantial spending on the related consequences of infection.

The infectious disease public health infrastructure, which carries out disease surveillance at the Federal, State, and local levels, is an essential tool in the fight against newly emerging and re-emerging infectious diseases. Other important defenses against infectious diseases include:

- Proper use of vaccines;
- Antibiotics;
- Screening and testing guidelines; and
- Scientific improvements in the diagnosis of infectious disease-related health concerns.

The Reproductive Health-Related Objective(s) are listed below.

- **IID-11 Increase routine vaccination coverage levels for adolescents IID.**

    - **IID-11.4 3 doses Human papillomavirus vaccine (HPV) for females by age 13 to 15 years**
        Data Source: National Immunization Survey (NIS) Teen, CDC, NCIRD, and NCHS

Baseline: 17 percent of females aged 13 to 15 years
                                    reported having been vaccinated with 3 or
                                    more doses of the human papillomavirus
                                    (HPV) vaccine in 2008
Target: 80 percent
Target-Setting Methodology: Consistency with national programs

Maternal, Infant, and Child Health

Goal
Improve the health and well-being of women, infants, children, and families.

Overview
Improving the well-being of mothers, infants, and children is an important public health goal for the United States. Their well-being determines the health of the next generation and can help predict future public health challenges for families, communities, and the health care system. The objectives of the Maternal, Infant, and Child Health topic area address a wide range of conditions, health behaviors, and health systems indicators that affect the health, wellness, and quality of life of women, children, and families.

Why Are Maternal, Infant, and Child Health Important?
Pregnancy can provide an opportunity to identify existing health risks in women and to prevent future health problems for women and their children. The risk of maternal and infant mortality and pregnancy-related complications can be reduced by increasing access to quality preconception (before pregnancy) and interconception (between pregnancies) care.[26] Moreover, healthy birth outcomes and early identification and treatment of health conditions among infants can prevent death or disability and enable children to reach their full potential.[27, 28, 29]

The Reproductive Health-Related Objective(s) are listed below.

- **MICH-16 (Developmental) Increase the proportion of women delivering a live birth who received preconception care services and practiced key recommended preconception health behaviors.**

    - **MICH-16.1 (Developmental) Discussed preconception health with a health care worker prior to pregnancy.**

Data Source:	Pregnancy Risk Assessment Monitoring System (PRAMS), CDC, NCCDPHP; California's Maternal and Infant Health Assessment (MIHA), Maternal, Child and Adolescent Health Department, California State Health Department
Baseline:	TBD
Target:	TBD
Target-Setting Method:	TBD

Maternal, Infant, and Child Health

- **MICH-17 Reduce the proportion of persons aged 18 to 44 years who have impaired fecundity (i.e., a physical barrier preventing pregnancy or carrying a pregnancy to term).**

  - **MICH-17.1 Reduce the proportion of women aged 18 to 44 years who have impaired fecundity.**

Data Source:	National Survey of Family Growth (NSFG), CDC, NCHS
Baseline:	12.0 percent of females aged 18 to 44 years had impaired fecundity in 2006-8
Target:	10.8 percent
Target-Setting Methodology:	10 percent improvement

  - **MICH-17.2 (Developmental) Reduce the proportion of men aged 18 to 44 years who have impaired fecundity.**

Data Source:	National Survey of Family Growth (NSFG), CDC, NCHS
Baseline:	TBD
Target:	TBD
Target-Setting Methodology:	TBD

Sexually Transmitted Diseases

Goal

Promote healthy sexual behaviors, strengthen community capacity, and increase access to quality services to prevent sexually transmitted diseases (STDs) and their complications.

Overview

STDs refer to more than 25 infectious organisms that are transmitted primarily through sexual activity. STD prevention is an essential primary care strategy for improving reproductive health.[30] Despite the fact that they are largely preventable, STDs remain a significant public health problem in the United States. STDs cause many harmful, often irreversible, and costly clinical complications, such as:

- Reproductive health problems;
- Fetal and perinatal health problems;
- Cancer; and
- Facilitation of the sexual transmission of HIV infection.[31]

Why Is Sexually Transmitted Disease Prevention Important?

The Centers for Disease Control and Prevention (CDC) estimates that there are approximately 19 million new STD infections each year—almost half of them among young people ages 15 to 24.[32] The cost of STDs to the U.S. health care system is estimated to be as much as $15.9 billion annually.[33] Because many cases of STDs go undiagnosed—and some common viral infections, such as human papillomavirus (HPV) and genital herpes, are not reported to CDC at all—the reported cases of chlamydia, gonorrhea, and syphilis represent only a fraction of the true burden of STDs in the United States.

Untreated STDs can lead to serious long-term health consequences, especially for adolescent girls and young women. The CDC estimates that undiagnosed and untreated STDs cause at least 24,000 women in the United States each year to become infertile.[34]

The Reproductive Health-Related Objective(s) are listed below.

- **STD-1 Reduce the proportion of adolescents and young adults with Chlamydia trachomatis infections.**

- o **STD-1.1 Among females aged 15 to 24 years attending family planning clinics**

Data Source:	STD Surveillance System (STDSS), CDC, NCHHSTP
Baseline:	7.4 percent of females aged 15 to 24 years who attended family planning clinics in the past 12 months tested positive for Chlamydia trachomatis infections in 2008
Target:	6.7 percent
Target-Setting Methodology:	10 percent improvement

- **STD-5 Reduce the proportion of females aged 15 to 44 years who have ever required treatment for pelvic inflammatory disease (PID).**

Data Source:	National Survey of Family Growth (NSFG), CDC, NCHS
Baseline:	3.99 percent of females aged 15 to 44 years reported that they had ever required treatment for pelvic inflammatory disease (PID), in 2006-8
Target:	3.59 percent
Target-Setting Methodology:	10 percent improvement

- **STD-6 Reduce gonorrhea rates.**

  - o **STD-6.1 Females aged 15 to 44 years**

Data Source:	STD Surveillance System (STDSS), CDC, NCHHSTP
Baseline:	285 new cases of gonorrhea per 100,000 females aged 15 to 44 years were reported in 2008
Target:	257 new reported cases per 100,000 population
Target-Setting Methodology:	10 percent improvement

- **STD-6.2 Males aged 15 to 44 years**

Data Source:	STD Surveillance System (STDSS), CDC, NCHHSTP
Baseline:	220 new cases of gonorrhea per 100,000 males aged 15 to 44 years were reported in 2008
Target:	198 new reported cases per 100,000 population
Target-Setting Methodology:	10 percent improvement

References

1. Institute of Medicine, Committee on Monitoring Access to Personal Health Care Services. Access to health care in America. Millman M, editor. Washington: National Academies Press; 1993.

2. Bierman A, Magari ES, Jette AM, *et al*. Assessing access as a first step toward improving the quality of care for very old adults. J Ambul Care Manage. 1998 Jul;121(3):17-26.

3. U.S. Census Bureau. 2008 population estimates: National characteristics, national sex, age, race and Hispanic origin. Washington: 2008. Available from: http://www.census.gov/popest/national/asrh/NC-EST2008-asrh.html

4. National Research Council and Institute of Medicine. Committee on Adolescent Health Care Services and Models of Care for Treatment, Prevention, and Healthy Development. Adolescent health services: Missing opportunities. Lawrence RS, Gootman JA, Sim LJ, editors. Washington: National Academies Press, 2009. Available from: http://books.nap.edu/openbook.php?record_id=12063&page=1

5. Mulye TP, Park MJ, Nelson CD, *et al*. Trends in adolescent and young adult health in the United States. *J Adolesc Health*. 2009;45(1):8-24. Available from: http://download.journals.elsevierhealth.com/pdfs/journals/1054-139X/PIIS1054139X09001244.pdf

6. National Research Council, Panel on High-Risk Youth, Commission on Behavioral and Social Sciences and Education. Losing generations: Adolescents in high-risk settings. Washington: National Academies Press; 1993. Available from: http://www.nap.edu/openbook.php?record_id=2113&page=1

7. McNeely C, Blanchard J. The teen years explained: A guide to healthy adolescent development. Baltimore: Johns Hopkins Bloomberg School of Public Health, Center for Adolescent Health; 2009. Available from: http://www.jhsph.edu/adolescenthealth

8. Halfon N, Hochstein M. Life course health development: An integrated framework for developing health, policy and research. Milbank Q. 2002;80(3):433-79. Available from: http://www.milbank.org/quarterly/8003feat.html 🖼

9. Gamm L, Castillo G, Williams L. Education and community-based programs in rural areas: A literature review. In: Rural Healthy People 2010: A companion document to Healthy People 2010, Volume 3. Gamm L, Hutchison L, editors. College Station, TX: The Texas A&M University System Health Science Center, School of Rural Public Health, Southwest Rural Health Research Center; 2004. p.167-86. Available from: http://www.srph.tamhsc.edu/centers/rhp2010/Volume_3/Vol3Ch4LR.pdf 🖼

10. Centers for Disease Control and Prevention. Achievement in public health, 1900–1999: Family planning. *MMWR Weekly*. 1999 Dec 3;48(47):1073-80.

11. Gold RB, Sonfield A, Richards C, et al. Next steps for America's family planning program: Leveraging the potential of Medicaid and Title X in an evolving health care system. New York: Guttmacher Institute; 2009.

12. US Department of Health and Human Services, Office of Public Health and Science, Office of Population Affairs, Office of Family Planning. Program guidelines for project grants for family planning services [Internet]. Bethesda, MD: Office of Family Planning; 2001 Jan [cited 2009 Apr 14]. Available from: http://www.hhs.gov/opa/familyplanning/toolsdocs/2001_ofp_guidelines_complete.pdf

13. Lindberg L, Frost J, Sten C, *et al.* Provision of contraceptive and related services by publicly funded family planning clinics, 2003. *Perspect Sex Reprod Health*. 2006 Sep;38(3):139-47.

14. Frost J. US women's reliance on publicly funded family planning clinics as their usual source of medical care. Paper presented at National Survey of Family Growth Research Conference; 2008 Oct.

15. Frost J, Finer L, Tapales A. The impact of publicly funded family planning clinic services on unintended pregnancies and government cost savings. *J Health Care Poor Underserved*. 2008 Aug;19(3):778-96.

16. Finer L, Henshaw S. Disparities in rates of unintended pregnancy in the United States, 1994 and 2001. *Perspect Sex Reprod Health*. 2006 Jun;38(2):90-6.

17. Trussell J. The cost of unintended pregnancy in the United States. Contraception. 2007 Mar;75(3):168-70.

18. Logan C, Holcombe E, Manlove J, *et al.* The consequences of unintended childbearing: A white paper [Internet]. Washington: Child Trends, Inc.; 2007 May [cited 2009 Mar 3]. Available from: http://www.childtrends.org/Files//Child_Trends-2007_05_01_FR_Consequences.pdf

19. Cheng D, Schwarz E, Douglas E, *et al.* Unintended pregnancy and associated maternal preconception, prenatal and postpartum behaviors. *Contraception*. 2009 Mar;79(3):194-8.

20. Kost K, Landry D, Darroch J. Predicting maternal behaviors during pregnancy: Does intention status matter? *Fam Plann Perspect*. 1998 Mar–Apr;30(2):79-88.

21. D'Angelo, D, Colley Gilbert B, Rochat R, et al. Differences between mistimed and unwanted pregnancies among women who have live births. *Perspect Sex Reprod Health*. 2004 Sep–Oct;36(5):192-7.

22. Centers for Disease Control and Prevention. HIV prevalence estimates—United States, 2006. MMWR. 2008;57(39):1073-76

23. Hall HI, Song R, Rhodes P, *et al.* Estimation of HIV incidence in the United States. JAMA. 2008;300(5):520-9

24. Marks G, Crepaz N, Janssen RS, *et al.* Estimating sexual transmission of HIV from persons aware and unaware that they are infected with the virus in the USA. AIDS. 2006;20(10):1447-50.

25. Centers for Disease Control and Prevention (CDC). Achievements in public health, 1900–1999: Control of infectious diseases. MMWR. 1999 Jul 30;48(29):621-9.

26. Centers for Disease Control and Prevention (CDC), Agency for Toxic Substances and Disease Registry (ATSDR). Recommendations to improve preconception health and health care—United States: A report of the CDC/ATSDR Preconception Care Work Group and the Select Panel on Preconception Care. Atlanta: CDC; 2006. 23 p. (MMWR Recomm Rep. 2006;55[RR-06]).

27. Centers for Disease Control and Prevention (CDC). Newborn screening for cystic fibrosis: evaluation of benefits and risks and recommendations for state newborn screening programs. Atlanta: CDC; 2004. 37 p. (MMWR Recomm Rep. 2004;53[RR-13]).

28. Centers for Disease Control and Prevention (CDC). Identifying infants with hearing loss—United States, 1999–2007. Atlanta: CDC; 2010. (MMWR. 2010;59[8]:220-3).

29. Watson MS, Mann MY, Lloyd-Puryear MA, *et al.*; American College of Medical Genetics, Newborn Screening Expert Group. Newborn screening: Toward a uniform screening panel and system [executive summary]. *Pediatrics.* 2006;117(5 Pt. 2):S296-307.

30. United Nations. Report of the International Conference on Population and Development, Cairo, Egypt, September 5–13, 1994. New York: United Nations; 1995.

31. St. Louis ME, Wasserheit JN, Gayle HD, editors. Janus considers the HIV pandemic: Harnessing recent advances to enhance AIDS prevention. *Am J Public Health.* 1997;87:10-12.

32. Weinstock H, Berman S, Cates W Jr. Sexually transmitted diseases among American youth: Incidence and prevalence estimates, 2000. *Perspect Sex Reprod Health.* 2004 Jan–Feb;36(1):6-10.

33. Chesson HW, Blandford JM, Gift TL, et al. The estimated direct medical cost of sexually transmitted diseases among American youth, 2000. Perspect Sex Reprod Health. 2004 Jan–Feb;36(1):11-9. [Review].

34. Centers for Disease Control and Prevention. Unpublished estimate